HOMEMADE MEXICAN COOKING

EASY & DELICIOUS HOMEMADE RECIPES!

By Delia Suarez

TABLE OF CONTENTS

Quick and Easy Mexican Chicken

Mexican Chicken

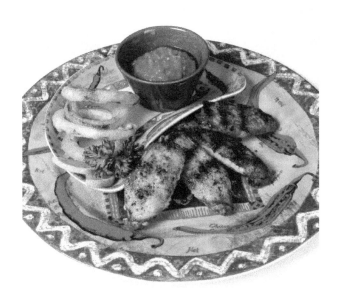

Ingredients

- 4 skinless, boneless chicken breasts
- 1 cup salsa
- 1 cup shredded Cheddar cheese 1 clove garlic, minced
- 1 pinch salt
- 1 pinch ground black pepper 1 pinch ground cumin

Directions

Preheat oven to 375 degrees F (190 degrees C).

Heat a greased skillet to medium. Rub chicken pieces with garlic, salt, pepper, and cumin to taste and add to hot skillet. Cook until brown on both sides and no longer pink (10 to 15 minutes).

Transfer meat to 9 x 13-inch baking dish or casserole dish, top with salsa and cheese, and bake at 375 degrees F (190 degrees C) for 15 to 20 minutes (until cheese is bubbly and starts to brown.) Serve over rice or buttered noodles.

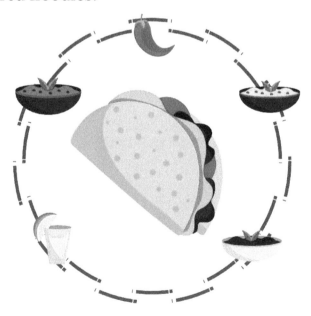

Mexican Chicken Kiev

Ingredients

- 8 skinless, boneless chicken breasts
- 2 green chile peppers, cut into
- 8 strips
- 1 (8 ounce) package Monterey Jack cheese, cut into 8 slices
- 1/2 cup butter, melted
- 1 cup Italian-style seasoned breadcrumbs
- 1 1/2 tablespoons grated Parmesan cheese
- 1/2 teaspoon salt
- 1/2 teaspoon ground cumin
- 1/2 teaspoon ground black pepper

Directions

Place 1 chicken breast between two sheets of wax paper. Working from the center to the edges, pound with a meat mallet until flat and rectangular shaped. Repeat with remaining breasts.

Wrap the green chili strips around the cheese, then wrap the flattened chicken breasts around the chili and cheese. Secure with toothpicks or uncooked spaghetti noodles.

Combine the breadcrumbs, parmesan cheese, salt, cumin, and pepper.

Roll the secured chicken pieces in the melted butter and then in the bread crumb mixture. Place chicken breasts in a 13x9 inch baking dish; don't let them, crowd. Drizzle the remaining butter over all eight of the breasts. Refrigerate for 1 hour, or freeze to bake later (baking time will be increased by about 5 to 10 minutes)

Bake in a preheated 400 degrees F (200 degrees C) oven for 25 to 30 minutes, or until chicken is no longer pink and juices run clear

Mexican Oxtail Beef Soup

Ingredients

- 2 tablespoons olive oil
- 2 pounds beef oxtail, cut into pieces
- 1-pound cubed beef stew meat (optional)
- 1 cube beef bouillon
- 1 onion, chopped
- 2 stalks celery, chopped
- 1/2 teaspoon chili powder
- 3/4 teaspoon ground cumin salt and pepper to taste
- 4 ears corn on the cob, broken in half
- 3 carrots, coarsely chopped
- 2 russet potatoes, cut into bite-sized pieces
- 1/3 cup lentils, picked over and rinsed
- 1/3 cup long-grain rice
- 1 cup frozen mixed vegetables (optional)
- 1 head cabbage, cored and cut into
- 8 wedges
- 8 corn tortillas (optional)

Directions

Heat the olive oil in a large soup pot over medium heat and brown the oxtails and beef stew meat on all sides. Add water to cover the meat, bring to a boil, reduce heat to a simmer, and cook for 30 minutes. Skim off and discard any foam that collects at the top.

Drop in the bouillon cube, onion, celery, chili powder, cumin, salt, pepper, and corn ears, stir to combine, and simmer the soup until the meat is very tender about 2 hours. Stir in the carrots and potatoes, simmer for 30 more minutes, then stir in the lentils, rice, mixed vegetables, and cabbage. Simmer until the rice, lentils, and cabbage are tender about 30 more minutes. Serve with a half ear of corn in each bowl, with hot steamed tortillas for dipping in the broth.

Mexican Zucchini Cheese Soup

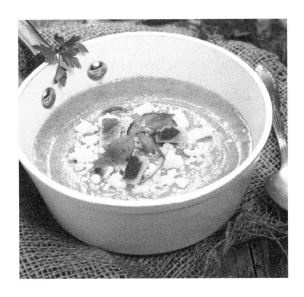

Ingredients

- 1 tablespoon olive oil
- 1 cup chopped onion
- 2 cloves garlic, minced
- 1/2 teaspoon dried oregano
- 2 (14.5 ounce) can chicken broth
- 1 (14.5 ounce) can Mexican-style stewed tomatoes
- 2 medium zucchinis, halved lengthwise and cut in 1/4-inch slices

- 2 medium yellow squash, halved lengthwise and cut in 1/4-inch slices
- 1 (8.75 ounce) can whole kernel corn, drained
- 1 (4.5 ounce) can diced green chile peppers
- 12 ounces processed cheese food, cubed
- 1/2 teaspoon freshly ground black pepper
- 1/4 cup chopped fresh cilantro

Directions

Heat the olive oil in a large pot, and saute the onion and garlic until tender. Season with oregano.

Mix in the chicken broth and tomatoes. Bring to a boil. Mix in the zucchini, yellow squash, corn, and chile peppers. Reduce heat to low, and simmer 10 minutes, or until the squash is tender.

Mix the cubed processed cheese into the soup. Continue to cook and stir until cheese is melted. Season with pepper. Mix in the cilantro just before serving.

Mexican Bean and Squash Soup

Ingredients

- 2 tablespoons olive oil
- 2 cups butternut squash - peeled, seeded, and cut into 3/4-inch chunks
- 1 small yellow onion, finely chopped
- 1/4 cup finely chopped celery
- 1/2 cup finely chopped carrot
- 3 cloves garlic, minced
- 2 canned Chipotle peppers in adobo sauce, seeded and minced 1 tablespoon chopped fresh basil leaves
- 1 tablespoon chopped fresh parsley
- 1 teaspoon cumin
- 1 (15 ounce) can diced tomatoes
- 2 quarts chicken broth
- 1 (15.5 ounce) can cannellini beans, drained
- 1 cup corn kernels, fresh, canned, or frozen
- 2 limes, cut into wedges
- 1 (10 ounce) bag tortilla chips for topping

- 1 cup sour cream for topping
- 1 (8 ounce) package shredded Mexican blend cheese for topping

Directions

Heat the olive oil in a deep pot over medium-high heat. Stir in the squash, and cook until it begins to soften 5 to 7 minutes. Add the onion, celery, and carrots. Cook until the onion is transparent, about 5 minutes. Stir in the garlic, chipotle peppers, basil, parsley, and cumin; cook 2 minutes more. Mix in the tomatoes and chicken broth. Reduce the heat to medium, and simmer until the vegetables are tender about 30 minutes. Stir in the cannellini beans and the corn; cook just until heated through.

To serve, ladle the soup into bowls. Squeeze lime juice over each bowl and top with tortilla chips, a dollop of sour cream, and a sprinkling of Mexican cheese.

Sopa De Lima (Mexican Lime Soup)

Ingredients

- 9 cups chicken broth
- 5 skinless, boneless chicken breast halves
- 1 large red onion, quartered
- 5 cloves garlic, chopped
- 2 teaspoons dried oregano
- 1 teaspoon salt
- 1 teaspoon ground black pepper
- 1/2 teaspoon dried thyme
- 1 tablespoon vegetable oil
- 4 green onions, chopped
- 1 large green chile pepper, seeded and chopped
- 2 large tomatoes, peeled and chopped
- 6 limes, juiced
- 1/2 lime
- 1/2 cup chopped fresh cilantro

Directions

Bring the chicken broth, chicken breasts, red onion, garlic, oregano, salt, pepper, and thyme to a boil in a large pot; reduce heat to medium-low and simmer until the chicken breasts are no longer pink in the center and the juices run clear 15 to 20 minutes. An instant-read thermometer inserted into the center should read at least 165 degrees F (74 degrees C). Remove the cooked chicken to a cutting board, shred into bite-sized strips; return to the simmering pot.

Heat the oil in a skillet over medium heat; cook the green onions and green chile pepper in the hot oil until tender, about 5 minutes. Stir the tomatoes into the mixture and continue cooking until soft, about 5 minutes more; pour the mixture into the pot with the chicken soup. Season with the salt; return the soup to a simmer. Add the lime juice and 1/2 a lime; cook another 10 minutes. Remove the pot from the heat and remove the lime half; stir in the cilantro to serve.

Mexican Chicken Soup

Ingredients

- 1/4 pounds skinless, boneless chicken breast halves
- 2 tablespoons taco seasoning mix
- 1 tablespoon vegetable oil
- 1/2 cup chopped onions
- 1/2 cup chopped celery
- 2 teaspoons ground cumin
- 1/4 teaspoon ground black pepper
- 1 cup water
- 3 (14 ounce) can chicken broth
- 1 cup diced tomatoes
- 1 tablespoon chopped fresh cilantro
- 1 cup shredded Cheddar cheese
- 1 cup crushed tortilla chips
- 1 avocado - peeled, pitted, and diced

Directions

Preheat oven to 350 degrees F (175 degrees C). Lay chicken breasts onto a baking sheet and sprinkle with 1 tablespoon taco seasoning mix. Bake for 30 to 35 minutes, cool, and shred or cut into strips.

While the chicken is cooking, heat oil in a stockpot and cook the onions and celery until soft. Stir in the water and chicken broth. Season with cumin, black pepper, and remaining taco seasoning mix. Simmer for 30 minutes for the flavors to mingle. Add the tomatoes, cilantro, and chicken, simmer for 5 more minutes. Serve hot topped with avocado, shredded cheese, and crushed tortilla chips.

Chili Mac, Mexican Style

Ingredients

- 2 fresh poblano chile peppers
- 1/2 tablespoon corn oil
- 1 pound chorizo sausage 1 medium onion, chopped
- 2 cloves garlic, minced
- 1 (28 ounce) can diced tomatoes with juice
- 1 (15 ounce) can black beans, rinsed and drained
- 1 cup water
- 1/2-pound macaroni
- 3/4 teaspoon salt, or to taste
- 1/4 teaspoon black pepper, or to taste
- 1/2 tablespoon dried Mexican oregano

Directions

Preheat oven to broil. Place peppers on a baking sheet and place in the oven. Allow skin to blacken and blister, turning the chile peppers until all sides are done. (Note: Do not overcook.) When they are done, place them in a paper bag and seal. In about 15 to 20 minutes, take them out of the bag and peel the skin off each one under running water. Remove the stems and seeds, then chop.

Heat oil in a Dutch oven over medium heat. Squeeze chorizo out of casings into the hot oil. With a wooden spoon, break up the sausage, and cook for about 4 minutes. Remove sausage and set aside. Stir onion into oil and cook until soft and translucent. Stir in garlic and cook for 1 minute. Stir in poblano peppers, and heat through 1 minute.

Increase the heat to high, and stir in tomatoes with liquid, black beans, water, macaroni, salt, pepper, and oregano. Bring to a low boil. Reduce heat to low; cover, and cook, occasionally stirring until the macaroni is al dente, about 10 minutes.

Jimmy's Mexican Pizza

Ingredients

- 1/2-pound ground beef
- 1 medium onion, diced 1 clove garlic, minced
- 1 tablespoon chili powder 1 teaspoon ground cumin
- 1/2 teaspoon paprika
- 1/2 teaspoon black pepper
- 1/2 teaspoon salt
- 1 (16 ounce) can refried beans
- 4 (10 inch) flour tortillas
- 1/2 cup salsa
- 1 cup shredded Cheddar cheese
- 1 cup shredded Monterey Jack cheese
- 2 green onions, chopped
- 2 roma (plum) tomatoes, diced
- 1/4 cup finely chopped jalapeno peppers
- 1/4 cup sour cream (optional)

Directions

Preheat the oven to 350 degrees F (175 degrees C). Coat 2 pie plates with non-stick cooking spray.

Place beef, onion, and garlic in a skillet over medium heat. Cook until beef is evenly browned. Drain off grease. Season the meat with chili powder, cumin, paprika, salt, and pepper.

Lay one tortilla in each pie plate, and cover with a layer of refried beans. Spread half of the seasoned ground beef over each one, and then cover with a second tortilla. Bake for 10 minutes in the preheated oven.

Remove the plates from the oven and let cool slightly. Spread half of the salsa over each top tortilla. Cover each pizza with half of the Cheddar and Monterey Jack cheeses. Place half of the tomatoes, half of the green onions, and half of the jalapeno slices onto each one.

Return the pizzas to the oven, and bake for 5 to 10 more minutes until the cheese is melted. Remove from the oven and let cool slightly before slicing each one into 4 pieces.

Mexican Turkey Burgers with Pico de Gallo

Ingredients

Pico de Gallo

- 3 medium tomatoes, chopped
- 1/3 cup chopped onion
- 2 cloves garlic, minced
- 1 serrano chile pepper, seeded and minced
- 1 lime, juiced
- 1/2 cup chopped fresh cilantro salt and pepper to taste

Turkey Burgers

- 1 pound ground turkey
- 1 egg
- 1/2 onion, minced
- 2 cloves garlic, minced
- 1 teaspoon ground coriander
- 1/2 teaspoon celery salt

- 1 teaspoon chili powder
- 1/2 teaspoon cumin
- 1 tablespoon chopped fresh parsley

Directions

In a bowl, mix together the tomatoes, the 1/3 cup chopped onion, 2 of the 4 cloves of minced garlic, serrano chile pepper, lime juice, and cilantro. Stir in salt and pepper to taste and set aside.

Place the ground turkey in a bowl. Add the egg, the 1/2 onion, minced, remaining 2 cloves minced garlic, coriander, celery salt, chili powder, cumin, and chopped parsley. Using your hands, work the mixture until all ingredients are evenly blended. Form mixture into 4 patties.

Heat a large, non-stick skillet for medium-high heat. Cook the turkey burgers for 5 minutes per side, or until no longer pink in the center and juices run clear. Reduce the heat as necessary during cooking. Serve with Pico de Gallo salsa.

Sweet Mexican Corn Cake

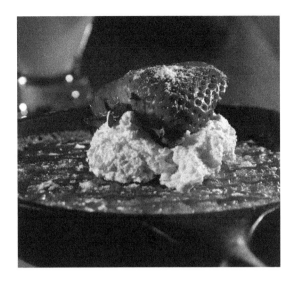

Ingredients

- 2 cups all-purpose flour
- 1 teaspoon baking powder
- 1 teaspoon ground cinnamon
- 1 teaspoon salt
- 1 1/4 cups unsalted butter, softened
- 1 cup white sugar
- 8 eggs
- 1 (14 ounce) can sweetened condensed milk
- 1 (12 fluid ounce) can evaporated milk
- 4 cups fresh corn kernels

Directions

Preheat an oven to 350 degrees F (175 degrees C). Grease and flour a 10x15-inch baking pan. Sift the flour, baking powder, cinnamon, and salt together into a bowl. Set aside.

Beat the butter and sugar together with an electric mixer in a large bowl until light and fluffy. Blend the eggs into the mixture one at a time. Stir the condensed milk and evaporated milk into the mixture. Add the flour mixture and mix until just incorporated. Fold the corn kernels into the batter, mixing just enough to evenly combine. Pour the batter into the prepared pan.

Bake in the preheated oven until a toothpick inserted into the center comes out clean, about 40 minutes. Cool in the pans for 10 minutes before removing to cool completely on a wire rack.

Mexican Wedding Cookies

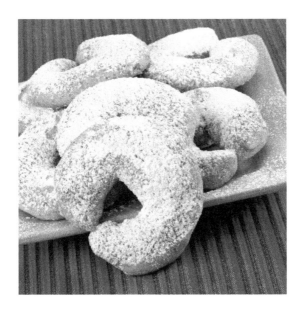

Ingredients

- 1 cup butter
- 1/2 cup white sugar
- 2 teaspoons vanilla extract
- 2 teaspoons water
- 2 cups all-purpose flour
- 1 cup chopped almonds
- 1/2 cup confectioners' sugar

Directions

In a medium bowl, cream the butter and sugar. Stir in vanilla and water. Add the flour and almonds, mix until blended. Cover and chill for 3 hours.

Preheat oven to 325 degrees.

Shape dough into balls or crescents. Place on an unprepared cookie sheet and bake for 15 to 20 minutes in the preheated oven. Remove from pan to cool on wire racks. When cookies are cool, roll in confectioners' sugar. Store at room temperature in an airtight container.

Mexican Shrimp Cocktail

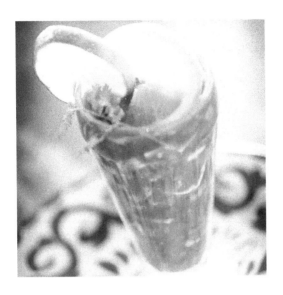

Ingredients

- 2 pounds cooked shrimp, peeled and deveined
- 1 tablespoon crushed garlic
- 1/2 cup finely chopped red onion
- 1/4 cup fresh cilantro, chopped
- 1 1/2 cups tomato and clam juice cocktail
- 1/4 cup ketchup
- 1/4 cup fresh lime juice
- 1 teaspoon hot pepper sauce, or to taste
- 1/4 cup prepared horseradish salt to taste
- 1 ripe avocado - peeled, pitted, and chopped

Directions

Place the shrimp in a large bowl. Stir garlic, red onion, and cilantro. Mix in tomato and clam juice cocktail, ketchup, lime juice, hot pepper sauce, and horseradish. Season with salt. Gently stir in avocado. Cover, and refrigerate for 2 to 3 hours. Serve in one large bowl or ladle into individual bowls.

Mexican Spaghetti Sauce

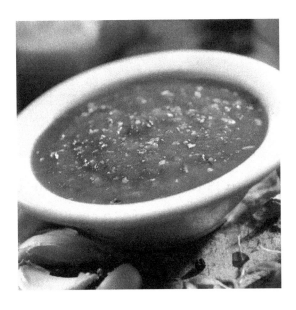

Ingredients

- 1 pound ground beef
- 3/4 cup chopped onion
- 4 cups hot water (150 degrees F to 160 degrees F)
- 1 (26 ounce) jar meatless spaghetti sauce
- 1 (15 ounce) can black beans, rinsed and drained
- 1 (14.5 ounce) can diced tomatoes 1 cup frozen corn, thawed
- 1 cup salsa
- 1 (4 ounce) can chopped green chilies

- 1 tablespoon chili powder
- 1/4 teaspoon salt
- 1/4 teaspoon pepper Hot cooked spaghetti

Directions

In a large nonstick, cook beef and onion over medium heat until meat is no longer pink, drain. Using a slotted spoon, remove beef mixture to several layers of white paper towels. Let stand for 1 minute. Blot top of the beef with additional white paper towels. Transfer beef mixture to fine mesh strainer over a 1-1/2-qt. bowl. Pour hot water over beef. Drain for 5 minutes.

In a large saucepan, combine spaghetti sauce, beans, tomatoes, corn, salsa, chilies, chili powder, salt, and pepper. Stir in beef mixture. Bring to a boil. Reduce heat; simmer, uncovered, for 10-15 minutes. Serve over spaghetti.

Mexican-Style Pork Chops

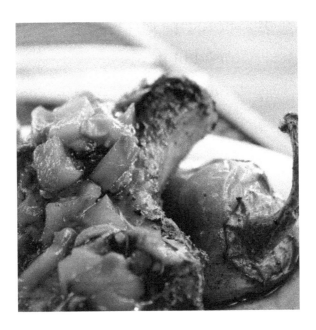

Ingredients

- 6 (1/2-inch thick) bone-in pork chops
- 2 tablespoons vegetable oil
- 1 medium onion, chopped
- 1 (16 ounce) can kidney beans, rinsed and drained
- 1 (15.25 ounce) can whole kernel corn, drained
- 1 (10.75 ounce) can condensed tomato soup, undiluted

- 1 1/4 cups water
- 1 cup uncooked instant rice
- 1/2 cup sliced ripe olives
- 2 teaspoons chili powder
- 1/2 teaspoon dried oregano 1/2 teaspoon salt
- 1/8 teaspoon pepper

Directions

In an ovenproof skillet, brown pork chops in oil on each side; remove and keep warm. In the same skillet, saute onion until tender. Stir in the remaining ingredients; bring to a boil. Place chops over the top. Bake, uncovered, at 350 degrees F for 35-40 minutes or until meat is tender.

Mexican Steak Torta

Ingredients

- 1 pound sirloin steak
- 1 tablespoon garlic salt
- 1 teaspoon ground black pepper
- 1 teaspoon ground cumin ground cayenne pepper to taste
- 4 kaiser rolls, split
- 1/4 cup mayonnaise
- 1/2 cup refried beans
- 1 large avocado, thinly sliced
- 1 large tomato, sliced
- 2 cups shredded lettuce crumbled cotija cheese (optional)

Directions

Preheat an outdoor grill for medium-high heat, and lightly oil the grate. Season steak with garlic salt, black pepper, cumin, and cayenne pepper.

Grill steak on the preheated grill until medium-rare, about 5 minutes per side. Remove from heat to a cutting board and cover with foil.

Set a large skillet over medium-high heat. Spread both halves of each roll with mayonnaise. Brown the rolls, mayonnaise-side down until golden, about 3 minutes. Warm the refried bean in a bowl in the microwave, about 1 minute on High, and slice the sirloin steak into thin strips.

Spread a thin layer of beans on the bottom half of each roll, layer with steak, avocado, tomato, and lettuce. Top with cheese, if desired, and close the sandwich with the top of the roll.

Mexican Hot Carrots

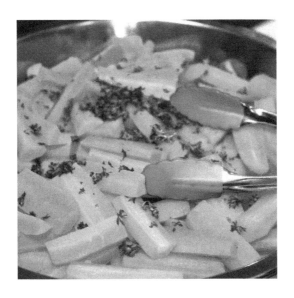

Ingredients

- 6 carrots, peeled and sliced
- 1 (16 ounce) jar sliced jalapeno peppers, with liquid
- 2 onions, thinly sliced
- 1 cup vinegar

Directions

Place the carrots in a saucepan with enough water to cover and cook over medium heat until nearly boiling, 7 to 10 minutes.

Immediately drain the carrots and set them aside to cool.

Divide the cooled carrots into two 1-quart glass jars. Alternate layers of onion and jalapeno peppers atop the carrots until the jars are full.

Mix the liquid from the jalapeno peppers and the vinegar in a saucepan; bring the mixture to a rolling boil. Remove from heat and pour the liquid into the jars until full. Seal the jars with lids. Place the jars in the refrigerator until cold, at least 8 hours.

Mexican Baked Fish

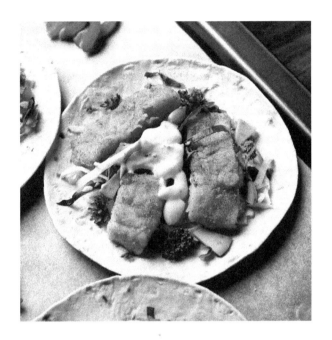

Ingredients

- 1 1/2 pounds cod
- 1 cup salsa
- 1 cup shredded sharp Cheddar cheese
- 1/2 cup coarsely crushed corn chips
- 1 avocado - peeled, pitted, and sliced
- 1/4 cup sour cream

Directions

Preheat oven to 400 degrees F (200 degrees C). Lightly grease one 8x12 inch baking dish.

Rinse fish fillets under cold water, and pat dry with paper towels. Lay fillets side by side in the prepared baking dish. Pour the salsa over the top, and sprinkle evenly with the shredded cheese. Top with the crushed corn chips.

Bake, uncovered, in the preheated oven for 15 minutes, or until fish is opaque and flakes with a fork. Serve topped with sliced avocado and sour cream.

Mexican Coffee

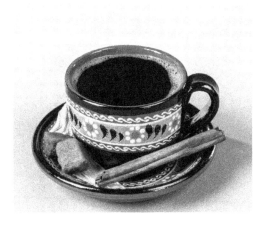

Ingredients

- 1 sugar cube
- 1 fluid ounce hot water
- 3/4 cup coffee
- 1 fluid ounce coffee-flavored liqueur
- 1 tablespoon whipped cream

Directions

Pour sugar and hot water into a coffee mug. Stir in the coffee and liqueur, and then spoon whipped cream gently on top of the coffee.

Mexican Steak and Beans

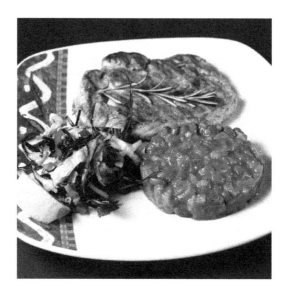

Ingredients

- 1 tablespoon all-purpose flour
- 1/2 teaspoon chili powder
- 1/4 teaspoon salt
- 1/8 teaspoon ground cumin
- 1/8 teaspoon pepper
- 1/2-pound boneless beef round steak, cut into 1-inch cubes
- 1 tablespoon vegetable oil
- 3/4 cup thinly sliced celery

- 1 medium onion, chopped
- 1/2 cup water
- 1/4 cup chili sauce
- 1 medium carrot, cut into
- 1/2-inch slices
- 1 small green pepper, cut into
- 1 1/2 -inch strips
- 3/4 cup kidney beans, rinsed and drained
- Hot cooked rice

Directions

In a resealable plastic bag, combine the first five ingredients. Add the steak; shake to coat. In a skillet, cook steak in oil until browned on all sides, drain. Add the celery, onion, water, and chili sauce.

Bring to a boil. Reduce heat; cover, and simmer for 30 minutes. Add carrot; cover, and simmer for 15 minutes. Stir in green pepper and beans. Cover and simmer 10 minutes longer or until meat and vegetables are tender. Serve over rice if desired.

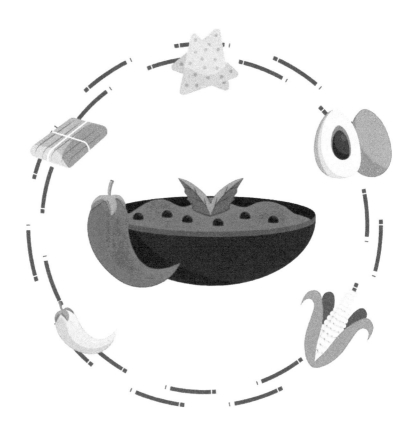

Mexican Shepherd's Pie

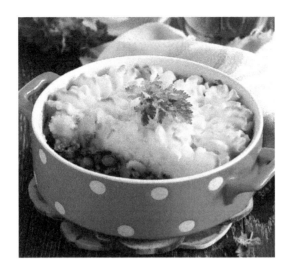

Ingredients

- 1 1/2 pounds ground beef
- 1 onion, finely chopped garlic powder to taste
- salt and pepper to taste
- 1 (14.5 ounce) can diced tomatoes
- 1 (1.25 ounce) package taco seasoning mix
- 3/4 cup hot water
- 1 (11 ounce) can whole kernel corn, drained
- 1 (8.5 ounce) package corn muffin mix
- 1 cup shredded Cheddar cheese (optional)
- 1 (2.25 ounce) can sliced black olives (optional)

Directions

Preheat oven to 400 degrees F (200 degrees C). Spray a 9x13 inch baking dish with cooking spray.

Place the beef and onion in a skillet over medium heat. Cook until beef is evenly brown and onion is tender. Drain grease. Season with garlic powder, salt, and pepper. Mix in the tomatoes and cook for 5 minutes. Stir in the taco seasoning and water. Bring to a boil, reduce heat to low, and continue cooking for 5 minutes until thickened. Transfer to the prepared baking dish, and top evenly with corn.

Prepare the corn muffin mix according to package directions. Spread evenly over the corn layer in the baking dish.

Bake 20 minutes in the preheated oven or until puffed and golden. Garnish with olives and cheese.

Mexican Pintos with Cactus

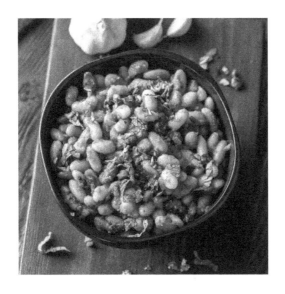

Ingredients

- 2 cups dry pinto beans, rinsed
- 3 tablespoons salt, divided
- 3 slices bacon, chopped
- 2 large flat cactus leaves (nopales)
- 1 jalapeno pepper, seeded and chopped
- 2 slices onion

Directions

Place the pinto beans into a slow cooker, and fill to the top with hot water. Add the bacon, 2 tablespoons of salt, jalapeno, and onion.

Cover, and cook on High for 3 to 4 hours, adding water as needed, until beans are tender.

Remove any thorns from the cactus leaves, and slice them into small pieces. Place in a saucepan with 1 tablespoon of salt, and fill with enough water to cover. Bring to a boil and cook for 15 minutes. Drain and rinse with cold water for 1 minute. Add to the beans when they are soft and cook for 15 more minutes on High.

Mexican Beef Supreme

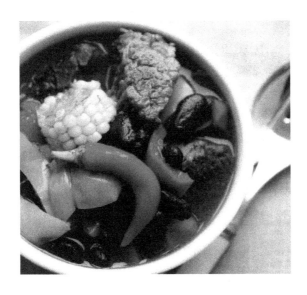

Ingredients

- 1 tablespoon olive oil
- 1 onion, diced
- 1-pound cubed beef stew meat
- 1 1/2 teaspoons minced garlic
- 1/2 lime, juiced
- 1 jalapeno pepper, seeded and chopped
- 3 green onions, chopped
- 1/4 cup chopped fresh cilantro, or to taste
- 1 teaspoon dried oregano
- 1 (7 ounce) can of green salsa

Directions

Heat olive oil in a large skillet over medium-high heat. Add the onion, and cook for a few minutes, then stir in the beef and garlic. Cook, frequently stirring until meat is evenly browned.

While the meat is cooking, stir together the lime juice, jalapeno, cilantro, and green onion. When the meat is browned, stir in the cilantro mixture and oregano. Pour in the salsa, cover, and cook for about 10 minutes, occasionally stirring, until the meat is cooked through.

Mexican Casserole

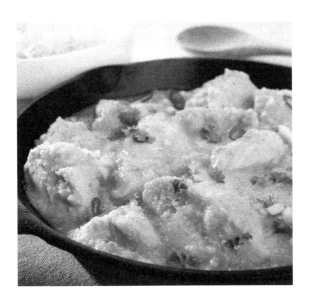

Ingredients

- 2 tablespoons vegetable oil
- 3/4-pound cubed skinless, boneless chicken breast meat
- 1/2 (1.25 ounce) package taco seasoning mix
- 1 (15 ounce) can black beans, rinsed and drained
- 1 (8.75 ounce) can sweet corn, drained
- 1/4 cup salsa water as needed
- 1 cup shredded Mexican-style cheese
- 1 1/2 cups crushed plain tortilla chips

Directions

In a large skillet over medium-high heat, saute chicken in oil until cooked through and no longer pink inside. Add taco seasoning, beans, corn, salsa, and a little water to prevent drying out. Cover skillet and simmer over medium-low heat for 10 minutes.

Preheat oven to 350 degrees F (175 degrees C).

Transfer chicken mixture to a 9x13 inch baking dish. Top with 1/2 cup of cheese and crushed tortilla chips.

Bake in the preheated oven for 15 minutes. Add remaining 1/2 cup cheese and bake until cheese is melted and bubbly.

Fideo (Mexican Spaghetti)

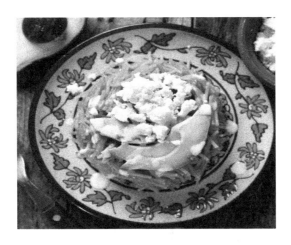

Ingredients

- 2 tablespoons vegetable oil
- 4 skinless, boneless chicken breast halves
- 1 (12 ounce) package spaghetti noodles, broken in half
- 5 roma (plum) tomatoes, chopped
- 1 large onion, chopped
- 1/2 tablespoon ground cumin
- 2 1/2 teaspoons chili powder salt and pepper to taste
- 1 1/2 cups water
- 1 cup shredded Cheddar cheese

Directions

Heat 1 tablespoon of vegetable oil in a large skillet over medium heat. Cook chicken breasts in the oil until nicely browned on the outside. Remove from the skillet and set aside.

Add remaining oil to the skillet and add the broken spaghetti. Cook, constantly stirring until spaghetti is browned. Drain off any excess oil and add tomatoes and onion. Dice the chicken breasts and return them to the skillet. Season with cumin, chili powder, salt, and pepper. Pour in water, cover, and simmer over medium-low heat until pasta is tender and water has been absorbed for about 10 minutes. Check towards the end and add more water if necessary.

Spoon the chicken mixture into bowls to serve, and garnish with shredded cheese.

Mexican Halibut Bake

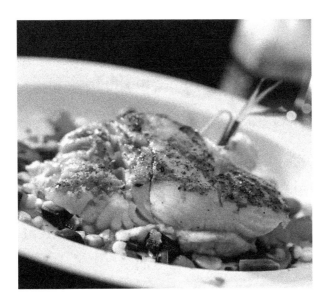

Ingredients

- 1/4 cup butter, melted
- 2 pounds skinless halibut fillets lemon pepper to taste
- 3/4 cup salsa
- 3/4 cup mayonnaise
- 3/4 cup sour cream
- 1 tablespoon garlic oil

Directions

Preheat oven to 350 degrees F (175 degrees C).

Pour the batter into the bottom of a baking dish. Arrange the halibut fillets in the dish and season with lemon pepper.

In a bowl, mix the salsa, mayonnaise, sour cream, and garlic oil. Spoon over the halibut fillets.

Bake halibut for 30 minutes in the preheated oven or until easily flaked with a fork.

Mexican Mango

Ingredients

- 1/4 cup water
- 1 tablespoon chili powder
- 1 pinch salt
- 3 tablespoons lemon juice
- 1 mango - peeled, seeded, and sliced

Directions

Bring water to a boil in a small saucepan. Stir in chili powder, salt, and lemon juice until smooth and hot. Add sliced mango and toss to coat; allow to soak up the chili sauce for a few minutes before serving.

Mexican Corn Bread

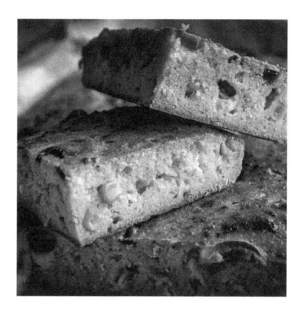

Ingredients

- 2 (8.5 ounce) packages corn bread/muffin mix
- 1 medium onion, chopped
- 2 cups shredded Cheddar cheese
- 1 (14.75 ounce) can cream-style corn
- 1 1/2 cups sour cream
- 4 eggs, beaten
- 1 (4 ounce) can chopped green chilies
- 1/3 cup vegetable oil
- 1 tablespoon finely chopped jalapeno pepper

Directions

In a bowl, combine cornbread mix and onion. Combine the remaining ingredients; add to the cornbread mixture just until moistened. Pour into a greased 13-in. x 9-in. x 2-in. baking dish. Bake at 350 degrees F for 50--55 minutes or until lightly browned and the edges pull away from the sides of the pan. Serve warm. Refrigerate leftovers.

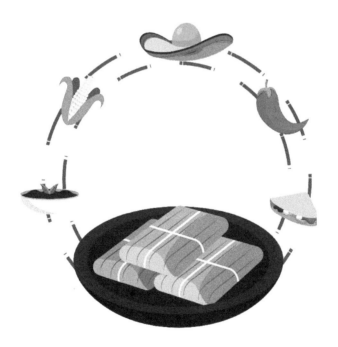

Mexican Sunset Bread

Ingredients

- 2/3 cup water (70 to 80 degrees F)
- 1/2 cup sour cream
- 3 tablespoons chunky salsa
- 2 1/2 tablespoons taco seasoning
- 4 1/2 teaspoons sugar
- 1 1/2 teaspoons dried parsley flakes
- 1 teaspoon salt
- 3 1/3 cups bread flour
- 1 1/2 teaspoons active dry yeast

Directions

In the bread machine pan, place all ingredients in the order suggested by the manufacturer. Select basic bread setting. Choose crust color and loaf size if available. Bake according to bread machine directions (check dough after 5 minutes of mixing; add 1 to 2 tablespoons of water or flour if needed).

Mexican Gump

Ingredients

- 1 cup dry macaroni
- 1 pound ground beef
- 1 small onion, chopped
- 1 (11 ounce) can whole kernel corn, drained
- 1 (10 ounce) can diced tomatoes with green chile peppers, drained
- 1 (1 pound) loaf processed cheese, cubed

Directions

Bring a pot of water to a boil. Add macaroni, and cook until tender, about 8 minutes. Drain.

While the macaroni is cooking, crumble the ground beef into a skillet over medium-high heat. Add the onion and cook and stir until browned. Drain off the grease. Reduce the heat to medium, and mix in the corn, tomatoes, cheese, and cooked noodles. Cook, stirring gently, until bubbly.

Marranitos (Mexican Pig-Shaped Cookies)

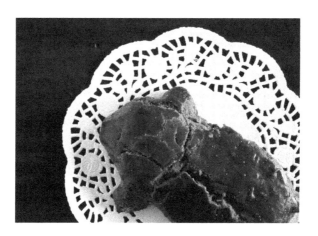

Ingredients

- 1 1/4 cups packed brown sugar
- 1/4 cup shortening
- 1 egg
- 1/4 cup milk
- 1 1/2 teaspoons vanilla extract
- 1 1/2 teaspoons baking soda
- 1 1/2 teaspoons ground cinnamon
- 1 cup unsulfured molasses
- 6 cups all-purpose flour
- 1 egg, beaten

Directions

Preheat the oven to 350 degrees F (175 degrees C). Line cookie sheets with parchment paper.

In a large bowl, cream together brown sugar and shortening until smooth. Mix in 1 egg, milk, and vanilla until smooth. Stir in the baking soda, cinnamon, and molasses. Mix in flour until the dough is stiff enough to roll out.

Roll dough out on a lightly floured surface to 1/4-inch thickness. Cut into cookies using a pig-shaped cookie cutter. Place cookies 2 inches apart on the prepared baking sheets. Brush the remaining beaten egg over the tops of the cookies.

Bake for 15 to 17 minutes in the preheated oven or until the centers of the cookies appear dry and edges are lightly browned.

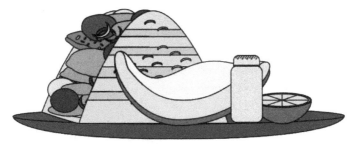

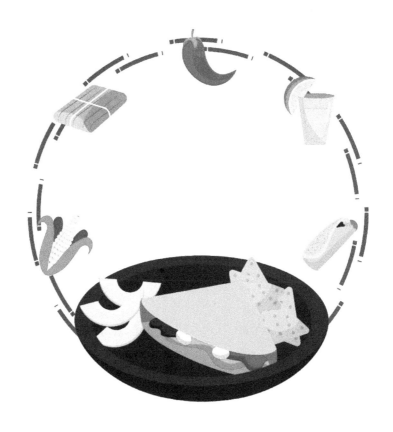

Mexican Sugar Cookies

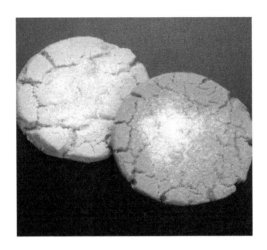

Ingredients

- 2 1/2 cups shortening
- 1 cup white sugar
- 1 teaspoon anise seed, ground
- 2 eggs
- 6 cups all-purpose flour
- 1 tablespoon baking powder
- 1/2 tablespoon cream of tartar
- 1/2 teaspoon salt
- 1/4 cup orange juice
- 3 tablespoons ground cinnamon
- 1 cup white sugar

Directions

Preheat oven to 350 degrees F (175 degrees C).

Beat shortening until light and fluffy. Add one cup of sugar and anise seed. Mix until creamy. Add eggs and mix well. Add flour, baking powder, cream of tartar, salt, and orange juice. Mix well.

Knead dough until smooth. On a lightly floured surface, roll to 1/2 inch thick. Cut using cookie cutter into different shapes. Bake until light brown, 5 - 8 minutes. Roll cookies in a mixture of 1 cup sugar and 3 tablespoons of cinnamon while still warm.

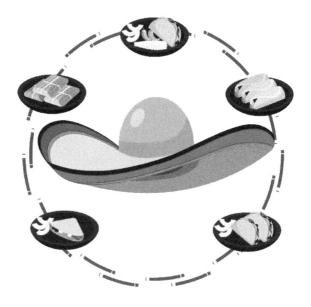

Mexican Cookie Rings

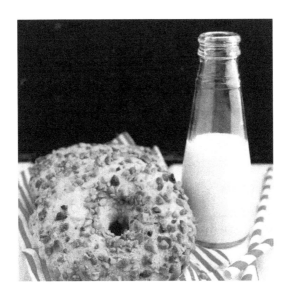

Ingredients

- 1 1/2 cups all-purpose flour
- 1/2 teaspoon baking powder
- 1/2 teaspoon salt
- 1/2 cup butter
- 2/3 cup white sugar
- 3 egg yolks
- 1 teaspoon vanilla extract
- 5 tablespoons multicolored sprinkles (jimmies) (optional)

Directions

Preheat oven to 375 degrees F (190 degrees C). Lightly grease baking sheets.

Sift together flour, baking powder and salt.

Cream together the butter and sugar. Add the egg yolks and vanilla, beating until light and fluffy. Mix in the dry ingredients.

Shape into 1-inch balls. Push your thumb through center of each ball and shape the dough into a ring. Dip top of each ring in decorating candies. Place cookies onto the prepared baking sheets.

Bake at 375 degrees F (190 degrees C) for 10 to 12 minutes or until golden brown. Remove from the baking sheets and let cool on racks.

Mexican Coffee Balls

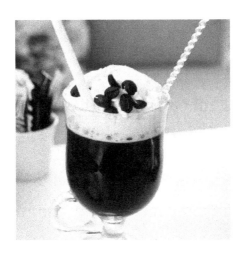

Ingredients

- 1 (9 ounce) package chocolate wafer cookies, crushed
- 1/2-pound ground almonds
- 1/3 cup unsweetened cocoa powder
- 1/4 cup white sugar
- 2 tablespoons instant coffee powder
- 1/3 cup coffee-flavored liqueur
- 1/2 cup light corn syrup
- 1/4 cup white sugar
- 2 teaspoons ground cinnamon

Directions

In a large bowl, mix chocolate wafer crumbs, ground blanched almonds, unsweetened cocoa powder, and 1/4 cup sugar.

Dissolve instant coffee in coffee liqueur and stir into crumb mixture with corn syrup.

Shape into 1/4-inch balls and roll in cinnamon sugar. To make cinnamon sugar, combine 1/4 cup sugar with 2 teaspoons cinnamon. Store in refrigerator.

Mexican Layered Dip

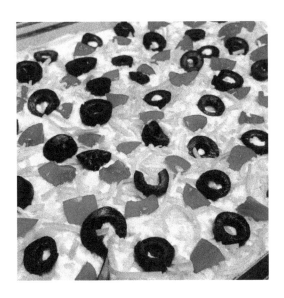

Ingredients

- 1 (16 ounce) can refried beans
- 1 (1.25 ounce) package taco seasoning mix
- 1 large tomato, seeded and chopped
- 1 cup guacamole
- 1 cup sour cream, room temperature
- 1 cup shredded sharp Cheddar cheese
- 1/2 cup chopped green onions
- 1/4 cup chopped black olives

Directions

Spread refried beans in the bottom of a (1-quart) shallow-edged serving dish (you can use a transparent dish if you'd like). Sprinkle the seasoning packet over the beans. Layer the diced tomatoes over the beans, the sour cream over the tomatoes, and the guacamole over the sour cream. Sprinkle the entire layered dip with cheddar cheese, followed by green onion, and finishing it off with a layer of black olives. Cover and refrigerate until ready to serve.

Mexican Green Chile Stew

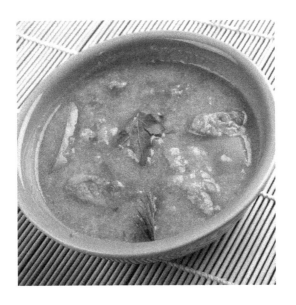

Ingredients

- 3 tablespoons olive oil
- 1 1/2 pounds beef chuck, cut into 1-inch cubes
- 1 1/2 pounds pork shoulder, cut into 1-inch chunks
- 1 green bell pepper, seeded and chopped
- 1 clove garlic, minced
- 2 (14.4 ounce) cans whole peeled tomatoes
- 1 (7 ounce) can chopped green chilies
- 1/3 cup chopped fresh parsley

- 1/2 teaspoon white sugar
- 1/4 teaspoon ground cloves
- 1/4 teaspoon ground cumin 1 cup dry red wine
- salt to taste

Directions

Heat the olive oil in a large skillet over medium heat. Cook and stir the beef and pork until evenly browned on all sides. Remove the meat using a slotted spoon and place in a bowl, then set aside.

Cook and stir the bell pepper and garlic in the same skillet until tender. Remove from heat.

Combine the tomatoes, green chiles, parsley, sugar, clove, cumin, and red wine in a large pot, breaking up the tomatoes using a spoon. Bring to a boil, then reduce heat to a simmer. Stir in the browned beef and pork along with their juice, then add the cooked green pepper and garlic. Cover and continue to cook over low heat for 2 hours, stirring occasionally. Remove lid and allow to simmer until sauce is reduced about 45 minutes.

Mexican Style Shredded Pork

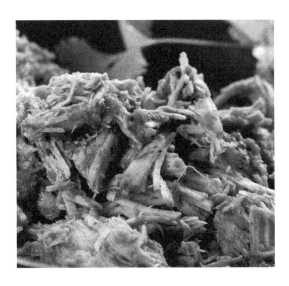

Ingredients

- 1 (3 pound) boneless pork loin roast, cut into 2-inch pieces
- 1/2 teaspoon salt
- 2 (4 ounce) cans diced green chile peppers
- 3 cloves garlic, crushed
- 1/4 cup chipotle sauce
- 3 1/4 cups water, divided
- 1 1/2 cups uncooked long-grain white rice
- 1/4 cup fresh lime juice
- 1/4 cup chopped cilantro

Directions

Place the roast in a slow cooker and season with salt. Place chile peppers and garlic on top of the roast. Pour in the chipotle sauce and 1/2 cup water.

Cover and cook 7 hours on Low.

In a pot, bring the remaining 2 3/4 cups of water and rice to a boil. Mix in the lime juice and cilantro. Reduce heat to low, cover, and simmer for 20 minutes.

Remove roast from the slow cooker and use two forks to shred. Return pork to the slow cooker and allow to sit 15 minutes to absorb some of the liquid. Serve over the cooked rice.

Mexican Venison Skillet

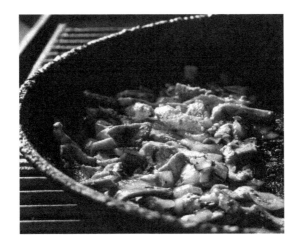

Ingredients

- 2 tablespoons butter or margarine
- 1 pound ground venison
- 2 teaspoons minced garlic 1 onion, chopped
- 2 tablespoons butter or margarine
- 1 (7 ounce) box Spanish rice mix
- 3 cups water
- 1 (14.5 ounce) can stewed tomatoes, cut up
- 1/2 cup salsa
- 1 (15.5 ounce) can kidney beans, rinsed and drained
- 1 (15.5 ounce) can sweet corn, drained

Directions

Melt butter in a large skillet over medium-high heat. Add venison and cook until no longer pink, stirring to break up. Stir in garlic and onion and continue cooking until the onion has softened and turned translucent for about 2 minutes.

Meanwhile, melt the remaining 2 tablespoons of butter in a saucepan over medium heat. Stir in Spanish rice mix, and cook until lightly golden, about 5 minutes. Stir in cooked venison, water, tomatoes, salsa, and kidney beans; bring to a boil, then reduce heat to medium-low and simmer for 15 minutes. Stir in corn, and continue cooking until the rice is tender about 5 minutes.

Pompous Mexican

Ingredients

- 1 (12 ounce) bottle Mexican beer
- 1/2 (1.5 fluid ounce) jigger full-flavored gin such as Tanqueray or Plymouth
- 3 tablespoons fresh lemon juice

Directions

Drink or pour out the beer to the level at which the neck widens, making room for the other ingredients. Pour in the gin and lemon juice. Secure the opening of the bottle using your thumb and gently rock the bottle to mix the ingredients. Drink and enjoy.

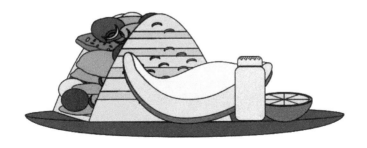

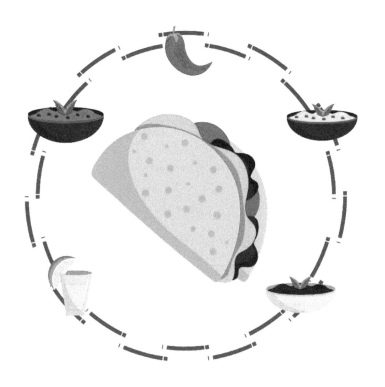

Slow Cooker Mexican Casserole

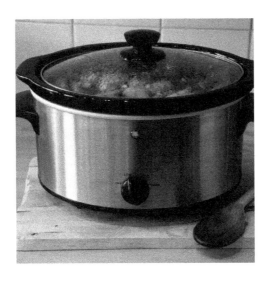

Ingredients

- 1 pound Bob Evans® Zesty Hot Sausage Roll
- 3/4 cup cornmeal
- 1 1/2 cups milk
- 1 egg
- 1 (14.5 ounce) can diced tomatoes and green chilies
- 1 cup frozen corn
- 1 (1.25 ounce) package taco seasoning mix
- 1 cup shredded Mexican blend cheese

Directions

Spray interior of slow cooker with non-stick vegetable spray. In a medium skillet over medium heat, crumble and cook sausage until brown. Place sausage in the slow cooker.

In a small bowl, combine cornmeal, milk, and egg. Stir into sausage. Add tomatoes, corn, and seasoning mix. Stir well. Cover and cook on low for 4 to 6 hours. Top with cheese 5 minutes before serving.

Recover to melt the cheese.

Mexican Chicken Salad

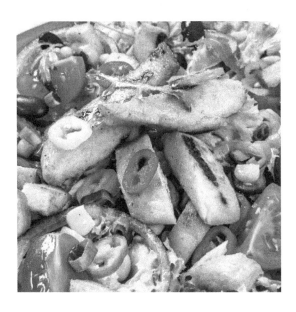

Ingredients

- 2 1/2 cups shredded cooked chicken meat
- 1/2 cup julienned carrots
- 1/4 cup julienned red bell pepper
- 1/4 cup julienned jicama
- 1/4 cup julienned red onion
- 2 (11 ounce) cans whole kernel corn, drained
- 1 cup cherry tomatoes, halved
- 3 avocados - peeled, pitted, and chopped
- 2 tablespoons chopped fresh cilantro

- 1/2 cup sour cream
- 2/3 cup mayonnaise
- 2 tablespoons fresh lemon juice
- 1/2 teaspoon ground cumin
- 1/2 teaspoon salt
- 1/4 teaspoon pepper
- 1 (1.25 ounce) package taco seasoning
- 1 teaspoon hot pepper sauce

Directions

In a large bowl, gently mix the chicken, carrots, red bell pepper, jicama, red onion, corn, cherry tomatoes, avocados, and cilantro.

In a separate bowl, mix the sour cream, mayonnaise, lemon juice, cumin, salt, pepper, taco seasoning, and hot pepper sauce. Pour over the salad and toss to coat. Cover and refrigerate at least 1 hour before serving.

Mexican Cheese Dip

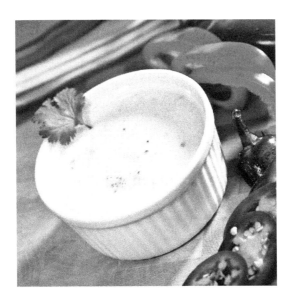

Ingredients

- 1 pound processed American cheese, cubed
- 1/2 pound fresh, ground spicy pork sausage
- 1 (12 ounce) package frozen chopped broccoli
- 1 (10 ounce) can diced tomatoes and green chiles

Directions

Place processed cheese spread in a microwave-safe bowl. Microwave on high in 2-minute increments (stirring at each pause) until the cheese spread is melted.

While the processed cheese spread is melting, brown sausage in a small skillet. Drain well.

Place broccoli in a microwave-safe bowl, cover, and microwave on high for 5 minutes.

In a large mixing bowl, combine melted cheese, sausage, broccoli, and diced tomatoes. Stir well before serving.

Mexican Beef and Bean Stew

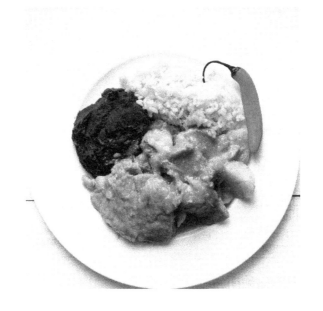

Ingredients

- 1/2 pounds beef for stew, cut in
- 1-inch pieces
- 2 tablespoons all-purpose flour 1 tablespoon vegetable oil
- 1 (10.5 ounce) can Campbell's® Condensed Beef Consommé
- 1 cup Pace® Thick & Chunky Salsa
- 1 large onion, coarsely chopped
- 1 (15 ounce) can pinto beans, rinsed and drained

- 1 (16 ounce) can whole kernel corn, drained
- 2 tablespoons chili powder 1 teaspoon ground cumin
- 1/4 teaspoon garlic powder

Directions

Coat the beef with flour. Heat the oil in a 12-inch skillet over medium-high heat. Add the beef and cook in 2 batches until it's well browned, stirring often.

Stir the beef, consommé, salsa, onion, beans, corn, chili powder, cumin, and garlic powder in a 3 1/2-quart slow cooker.

Cover and cook on LOW for 8 to 9 hours* or until the beef is fork-tender.

Mexican Stir-Fry

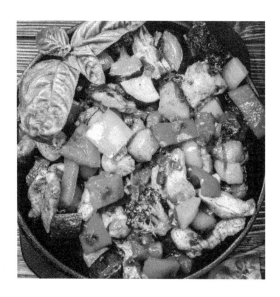

Ingredients

- 1/2 cup chopped onion
- 2 garlic cloves, minced
- 2 teaspoons vegetable oil
- 1/2 cup finely chopped green pepper
- 1/2 cup finely chopped sweet red pepper
- 2 tablespoons minced jalapeno pepper
- 3/4 cup water
- 1/2 cup tomato puree
- 1/2 teaspoon chili powder

- 1/2 teaspoon chicken bouillon granules
- 1/4 teaspoon salt
- 1 pinch cayenne pepper
- 1 1/3 cups diced cooked chicken
- 2/3 cup canned kidney beans, rinsed and drained
- 1 cup cooked rice
- 1/2 cup shredded Cheddar cheese

Directions

In a large skillet, saute onion and garlic in oil for 3 minutes. Add peppers; saute until crisp-tender, about 2 minutes. Stir in water, tomato puree, chili powder, bouillon, salt, and cayenne; bring to a boil. Reduce heat; simmer, uncovered, for 5 minutes. Add chicken, beans, and rice, heat through. Sprinkle with cheese.

Mexican Bean and Rice Salad

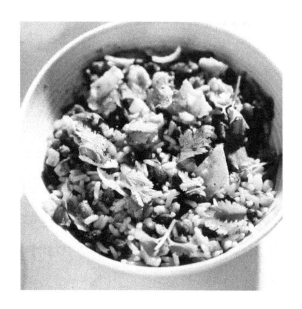

Ingredients

- 2 cups cooked brown rice
- 1 (15 ounce) can kidney beans, rinsed and drained
- 1 (15 ounce) can black beans, rinsed and drained
- 1 (15.25 ounce) can whole kernel corn, drained
- 1 small onion, diced
- 1 green bell pepper, diced
- 2 jalapeno peppers, seeded and diced
- 1 lime, zested and juiced

- 1/4 cup chopped cilantro leaves 1 teaspoon minced garlic
- 1 1/2 teaspoons ground cumin salt to taste

Directions

In a large salad bowl, combine the brown rice, kidney beans, black beans, corn, onion, green pepper, jalapeno peppers, lime zest and juice, cilantro, garlic, and cumin. Lightly toss all ingredients to mix well, and sprinkle with salt to taste.

Refrigerate salad for 1 hour, toss again, and serve.

Bekki's Mexican Egg Rolls

Ingredients

- 2 tablespoons vegetable oil
- 1 pound ground beef
- 1 large onion, chopped
- 5 cloves garlic, minced
- 1 red bell pepper, chopped
- 1 (1 ounce) package taco seasoning
- 1 (8 ounce) jar taco sauce
- 4 (16 ounce) packages egg roll wrappers
- (1 pound) loaf processed cheese food (i.e., Velveeta®), cut into 1/4-inch-thick slices
- 2 egg whites, lightly beaten
- 2 quarts canola oil

Directions

Place the vegetable oil and ground beef into a large skillet; cook over medium-high heat until the meat is evenly browned and no longer pink. Reduce the heat to medium. Mix in the onion, garlic, and bell pepper; cook until the vegetables are softened, about 5 minutes. Stir in the taco seasoning and taco sauce. Continue to cook and stir the mixture until the sauce begins to bubble, about 5 minutes more.

Working on a clean, flat surface, place 1 egg roll wrapper with a corner facing you. Place 1 tablespoon of the meat mixture in the center of the wrapper and top with a slice of cheese. Fold the corner closest to you over the meat mixture and roll the wrapper over the mixture 1-1/2 times. Fold in the two opposite side corners and continue rolling the wrapper, so it covers these corners, tucking them in. Dip two fingers in the egg whites and brush the remaining corner, pressing it to seal. Repeat these steps with a second egg roll wrapper. Let the egg roll rest briefly, so the egg white dries and holds the last corner in place.

If the egg rolls are not served right away, preheat the oven to 325 degrees F (165 degrees C). Line a heat-proof dish with paper towels.

Pour the canola oil into a large wok set over medium-high heat. When the oil begins to shimmer, carefully slip two to three egg rolls into the wok. Cook until the wrappers turn golden brown and bubble slightly, 30 seconds to 1 minute. Use a slotted spoon or strainer to remove from the wok. Place the egg rolls in the prepared dish and put the dish in the heated oven, making sure to remove it after 15 minutes or lower the temperature. Continue cooking the remaining egg rolls.

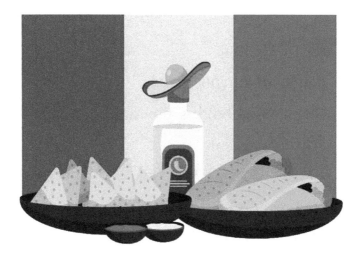

Authentic Mexican Tortillas

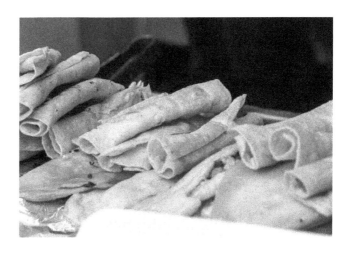

Ingredients

- 3 cups all-purpose flour
- 2 teaspoons baking powder
- 2 teaspoons salt
- 3/4 cup shortening
- 3/4 cup hot water

Directions

Combine the flour, baking powder, and salt. Either by hand or with a pastry cutter, cut in the shortening till the mixture is crumbly. If the mixture looks more floury than crumbly, be sure to add just one or two more tablespoons of shortening till it is crumbly. Add about 3/4 cup hot water to the mixture, or just enough to make the ingredients look moist.

With your hand or a large fork, knead the mixture making sure to rub the dough against the sides of the large mixing bowl to gather any clinging dough. If the dough still sticks to the side of the bowl, add a couple more tablespoons of flour until the dough forms a soft round shape. The dough is ready to roll out now, but it is best to let it rest. Cover it with a dishtowel, and let it sit for about an hour or so.

Take the dough and pull it apart into 10 to 12 balls. Lightly flour your rolling area and roll each ball with a rolling pin to about 1/8-inch thickness.

Place each tortilla on a medium-hot cast-iron skillet. Cook for about 1 to 2 minutes on each side or until the tortilla does not look doughy.

Mexican Pasta

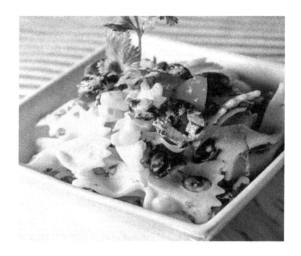

Ingredients

- 1/2-pound seashell pasta
- 2 tablespoons olive oil
- 2 onions, chopped
- 1 green bell pepper, chopped
- 1/2 cup sweet corn kernels
- 1 (15 ounce) can black beans, drained
- 1 (14.5 ounce) can peeled and diced tomatoes
- 1/4 cup salsa
- 1/4 cup sliced black olives
- 1 1/2 tablespoons taco seasoning mix
- salt and pepper to taste

Directions

Bring a large pot of lightly salted water to a boil. Add pasta and cook for 8 to 10 minutes or until al dente; drain.

While pasta is cooking, heat olive oil over medium heat in a large skillet. Cook onions and pepper in oil until lightly browned, 10 minutes. Stir in corn and heat through. Stir in black beans, tomatoes, salsa, olives, taco seasoning, and salt and pepper and cook until thoroughly heated, 5 minutes.

Toss sauce with cooked pasta and serve.

CPSIA information can be obtained
at www.ICGtesting.com
Printed in the USA
LVHW080037050621
689455LV00020B/1241